# The Metabolism Reset Diet Book

Reset Your Metabolism & Get Your Dream Body
in Just 30 days incl. 30 Days Weight Loss Challenge

## [1. Edition]

## Alan Roger Parker

# CONTENTS

**Introduction** ............................................................................................1

Metabolism ...............................................................................................1

What is the metabolism reset diet? ...........................................................3

Where do I have to pay attention?.............................................................4

    Physical Activities...............................................................................4

    Drinking Water....................................................................................4

    Sleep Cycle .........................................................................................5

    Lowered Stress Level ......................................................................... 6

Advantages of the Metabolism Reset Diet ................................................7

    Liver Health.........................................................................................7

    Weight Loss.........................................................................................7

    Blood Sugar Control .......................................................................... 8

Preparation ............................................................................................. 9

    Consult with a Dietician ................................................................... 9

    Hire a Personal Trainer..................................................................... 9

    Keep a Food Log................................................................................ 9

    Set Rewards for Milestone Achievements .......................................10

    Create a Support Network ...............................................................10

**Recipes**................................................................................................11

Breakfast (10 Recipes) ........................................................................... 13

    Berry Blast........................................................................................ 14

    Almond and Bacon Pancakes ......................................................... 15

    Breakfast Burrito ............................................................................. 16

    Blueberry Muffin Parfait ................................................................. 18

    Baked Ham and Cheese ...................................................................20

Boiled Eggs and Sweet Potatoes .................................................. 21

Quinoa Porridge ....................................................................22

Apple Tea...........................................................................23

PBJ Oatmeal Cups ................................................................. 24

Light Smoothie .................................................................... 25

Lunch Recipes.......................................................................27

BBQ Chicken Salad ................................................................ 28

Chicken Lettuce Wraps ........................................................... 29

Miso Beef Ramen.................................................................. 31

Radish and Asparagus Salad ....................................................33

Veggie Tabbouleh.................................................................. 34

Double-Cooked Potato Skins....................................................35

Bean Tacos with Green Salsa ....................................................37

Black Bean Soup................................................................... 39

Tijuana Torta.......................................................................40

Zucchini Chili-Cheddar Mash.................................................... 41

Dinner Recipes..................................................................... 43

Turkey Skewers with Coconut ................................................... 44

Chicken Breasts with Almond Cream Sauce .................................. 45

Baked Shrimp Enchilada..........................................................47

Beef Bean Verde....................................................................48

Pork and Soba Noodles...........................................................49

Chicken Noodle Soup.............................................................. 51

Tamarind Fish and Okra .......................................................... 53

Taco Meatloaf...................................................................... 55

Chicken Chili Rellenos ............................................................56

Salmon with Mango Sauce.................................................................57

Snacks & Desserts.............................................................................59

Berry Lemonade Sorbet ..................................................................60

Beef Chimichangas...........................................................................61

Mango Ceviche with Scallops.........................................................63

Apple Cheesecakes...........................................................................64

Pepper and Paprika Soup ...............................................................65

**30-Day Weight Loss Plan** ............................................................. **67**

Introduction ......................................................................................68

DAY 1 ....................................................................................................69

DAY 2 ...................................................................................................70

DAY 3 .....................................................................................................71

DAY 4 ....................................................................................................72

DAY 5 ....................................................................................................73

DAY 6 ....................................................................................................74

DAY 7.....................................................................................................75

DAY 8 ...................................................................................................76

DAY 9 .....................................................................................................77

DAY 10 .................................................................................................78

DAY 11 ...................................................................................................79

DAY 12 ..................................................................................................80

DAY 13 ....................................................................................................81

DAY 14 ..................................................................................................82

DAY 15...................................................................................................83

DAY 16...................................................................................................84

DAY 17 ........................................................................................... 85

DAY 18 ........................................................................................... 86

DAY 19 ........................................................................................... 87

DAY 20 ........................................................................................... 88

DAY 21 ........................................................................................... 89

DAY 22 ........................................................................................... 90

DAY 23 ........................................................................................... 91

DAY 24 ........................................................................................... 92

DAY 25 ........................................................................................... 93

DAY 26 ........................................................................................... 94

DAY 27 ........................................................................................... 95

DAY 28 ........................................................................................... 96

DAY 29 ........................................................................................... 97

DAY 30 ........................................................................................... 98

**Disclaimer** ............................................................................... **99**

**Imprint** ..................................................................................... **101**

# Metabolism

In the simplest terms, metabolism is the process through which the food items you eat or drink are converted into energy. This process basically consists of multiple chemical reactions which help in breaking down the original food particles. It is a complicated biochemical method which we, as well as other living beings, require to continue survival.

Our body performs a large array of crucial functions on a daily basis which we often don't pay any attention to. Such functions include breathing, blood circulation, growing cells and adjusting hormonal levels. They continue to perform even when we are sleeping. As a result, each of them demands a significant amount of energy that can be received from food.

Calories we intake are converted to energy by the metabolism process so that we can stay alive. The rate at which our body actively burns calories is called the metabolic rate, while the rate at which it burns calories at rest is called the basal metabolic rate or BMR. The design of your metabolism reset regimen will depend quite a lot on this BMR.

There is an ideal BMR for every human. This number depends on the size, gender, age, body temperature and hormonal production of that human. You can either determine your ideal BMR through a lab test or use the Harris-Benedict Equation for it. This equation applies to men and women differently as follows:

*Men's BMR = 88.362 + (12.397 x weight in kg) + (4.8 x height in cm) - (5.677 x age in years)*

*Women's BMR = 447.593 + (9.247 x weight in kg) + (3.098 x height in cm) - (4.33 x age in years)*

These are the factors which are not usually in our control. Therefore, we must focus on the other two factors contributing to our metabolic rate - exercises and food intake. By taking the right nutrients in the right amount and investing time in daily physical activities, one can attain a much higher metabolic rate. For example, drinking caffeine can function as a stimulant in increasing metabolism.

Along with converting food to energy, metabolism also helps to build blocks of several crucial components (like protein, nucleic acid, lipid, etc.) and to get rid of nitrogenous wastes.

# What is the metabolism reset diet?

One of the main reasons we are even talking about metabolism is its potential effect on weight loss. It is a common belief that people who have a fast metabolism can digest and process the food faster. As a result, their body tends to prevent excess calories from staying in the body.

However, the reality is that you can blame metabolism to a small extent when it comes to weight gain or loss. Metabolism is only responsible for regulating the breakdown of nutrient chemicals in your body to result in required energy.

The actual process of gaining or losing body weight is much more complex than just resetting metabolism. You need the right dietary habits, sleep cycle, exercise routine, hormonal controls, genetic composition and low stress level to reach the optimum weight effectively. The one aspect you should control is not eating more calories than your body can burn, because this is precisely what leads to unnecessary weight gain.

If you have figured out how to incorporate these factors into your weight loss mission, you can rely on the metabolism reset diet to work properly. You can use this diet to increase the metabolic rate of your body and thus make it burn more calories. It greatly helps with repairing the liver, optimizing thyroid and avoiding fat storage in your body.

This diet plan focuses on fruits, dairy and whole grain Ingredients to boost metabolism. You can follow it for 1 or 2 months according to your individual requirements.

# Where do I have to pay attention?

Along with taking the right food on a daily basis, you also need to focus on other factors to drive the metabolic rate higher. You must commit to the following for the 30 days of your diet for it to work effectively:

## Physical Activities

High metabolism is usually the result of many aspects out of our control like gender, age and genetic code. However, we can bring significant changes to our body's metabolic rate by investing long hours of rigorous exercises.

Muscle cells help in burning calories more efficiently than fat cells. When your workout session is over and your body has stopped sweating, these cells still stay in action to break down calories. The older people require to do more exercises since the muscle mass starts to decrease with age. As a result, the metabolism process also slows down with growing age. Daily physical activities can prevent this downfall.

Aerobic exercises like Zumba help the most in burning calories. You can make it even more efficient by switching between the intensity levels. Mix up the different exercise forms to take advantage of the switch. For instance, do jumping jacks for 1 minute and then walk for a couple of minutes. Feel free to take intervals in order to reach your maximum potential. You can also lift weights twice a week.

## Drinking Water

Keeping your body hydrated can increase its metabolism. Both hydration and metabolism are crucial to our survival. These two processes help to reach and maintain the optimum efficiency of your body. Hydration helps in restoring glucose transport and increasing their insulin sensitivity. If your body is lacking in water, it will slow down your metabolism and thus burn less calories. As a result, more fat will get the chance to stay increasing your overall weight.

Replace the usual soft drinks you take with cold water. Drinking half a liter of water will lift up your basal metabolic rate by up to 30% for one hour. Most dieticians recommend drinking cold water instead of hot water since it functions as a catalyst in burning lot of energy. The cold water is transformed into hot water using the reserved energy.

Water can help in keeping the weight off by making you feel full. Drink half a liter glass of water 30 minutes before eating and you will tend to consume less than usual. Adult subjects of a 2009 study successfully lost 44% more weight by drinking water this way.

## Sleep Cycle

It is essential to get a sound uninterrupted sleep every night. In order to regulate metabolism, sleep is extremely important for mammalians like humans. Our sleep has two distinct stages called REM and non-REM. The latter phase of sleep carries great value in maintaining metabolism.

The two main processes of metabolism are anabolism and catabolism. The first helps in building molecules while the latter breaks them down. Both of these processes function more efficiently during the non-REM sleep phase. This helps the body overcome the metabolic damages which occurred during their awake hours.

Not getting enough sleep will cause your metabolism to be unbalanced and enforce your body to crave for more carbohydrates. As a result, you can gain more weight. A 2011 study by Matthew Walker has shown that in the last six decades, the average number of sleeping hours has decreased, causing a rise of 10% to 23% in obesity.

Sleep deprivation can also lead to type 2 diabetes which can be prevented by investing in a metabolism reset diet. It can change hormone production and reduce thyroid secretion. So try your best to get 8 hours of sleep every night at minimum.

## Lowered Stress Level

Try your best to eliminate the possibilities of stress in your daily life. A high level of stress can result in the production of the hormone Cortisol. It is known to overtake multiple hormones and hamper glucose formation resulting in triggering obesity. Besides, anti-stress hormones like norepinephrine also pushed down the metabolic rate.

Along with low metabolism, these hormones can also cause high blood pressure, lipid disorders and type 2 diabetes in the long-term. You can attempt to lower the stress levels by practicing deep breathing and yoga. Regular exercise, healthy sleep cycle, keeping a journal, soothing music, green tea and certain supplements can also help with such a situation.

# Advantages of the Metabolism Reset Diet

This diet definitely increases your metabolism and helps you enjoy a much healthier lifestyle. However, by switching to the metabolism reset diet, you can also benefit from the following advantages:

## Liver Health

Liver is the main metabolic organ in the human body. It is responsible for regulating fat, carbohydrate and protein. The liver cells help to break down fats and give body the essential amount of energy. Irregularities involved in liver functionalities can result in harmful diseases like NAFLD (non-alcoholic fatty liver disease). It is a major cause behind triggering obesity.

Metabolism reset diet can fix such issues of the liver by reducing the amount of fat stored there. You can benefit from equal or higher levels of energy in daily life by switching to this diet.

## Weight Loss

One of the best effects of metabolism reset diet is its capability to reduce body fat while still maintaining lean mass. A major portion of this diet consists of whole foods. As a result, your body will receive a lot more fiber than usual. Such high fiber intake can help you on the weight loss mission.

The food items included in metabolism reset diet are generally much lighter. Thus your body will automatically get used to low calorie consumption. If you can pair this diet with weekly exercise routine, you can lose weight and gain healthy muscle mass simultaneously. Keep hydration in mind while investing in physical activities.

A downside is that the lost weight can be regained very easily when you leave this diet. You can keep the weight at or under optimum level for up to two months on this diet.

## Blood Sugar Control

This diet focuses on increased fiber intake much more than the other diets. Such an increase in the soluble fiber results in higher insulin sensitivity and glycemia improvement. As a result, it becomes easier for your body to control blood sugar levels. This, in turn, ensures a reduced possibility of type 2 diabetes. It also helps to prevent constipation, gastroesophageal reflux disease and hemorrhoids.

Increased Strength

Since metabolism reset diet helps in retaining muscle mass, it can also help you grow stronger even while reducing fat. The variety of wholesome food items in your diet will make it easier for the body to stay strong. It gets to function in an anabolic environment which helps with the increased strength.

# Preparation

Before starting to follow the metabolism reset diet, you can take the following steps in order to magnify and sustain the benefits:

## Consult with a Dietician

Consult with a trusted dietician to figure out the intricate details of your diet plan. She can help you to understand the potential side-effects and if it is the right diet for your individual health conditions. A dietician can also help you to figure out how to adapt your current lifestyle to this new diet. As a result, it will get easier for you to follow the strict diet rules for the 30 days.

## Hire a Personal Trainer

If you are not accustomed to exercises or routine physical activities in general, invest in a personal trainer to teach you how to do that. Remember that skipping or ignoring exercises will render the diet almost useless. You must set different milestones in order to maintain the weight loss rate and sustain the optimum muscle mass. A personal trainer can help you in this regard by pushing and motivating you to do your best.

## Keep a Food Log

No matter what you eat, record it somewhere. It could be a notebook or a mobile app - whatever you prefer. But keeping a log of your daily diet is essential to identify if you are improving or going backward. Track the changes and figure out with your dietician how to make it better for yourself.

## Set Rewards for Milestone Achievements

If you have successfully achieved a milestone in weight loss, give yourself something nice in return. This should not be some dessert or pizza from your favorite bakery. It should instead be a shopping spree, a massive concert or a relaxing pedicure. Rewarding yourself will increase your own motivation into building the life and body you have always dreamt of.

## Create a Support Network

We often tend to undermine the significance of a support network. A bunch of supportive friends and family can take you a lot further in your weight loss mission. If they are not available, join an online group or local community of people like you who are striving to lose weight. You can keep inspiring each other to achieve the individually set goals.

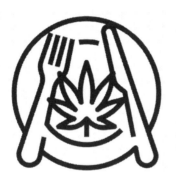

**Time: 1 hour 10 minutes | Serves 4**

Net carbs: 70% (21g/0.74oz) | Fiber: 13% (4g/0.14oz) | Fat: 3% (1g/0.03oz)

Protein: 10% (3g/0.1oz) | Kcal: 109

## Ingredients:

- 2 cups ice
- ⅓ cup of different berries
- 1 sliced orange
- 1 quartered lime
- Water as per need

## Preparation:

| | |
|---|---|
| **1.** | Place the orange slices and lime pieces in a large pitcher. |
| **2.** | Add the berries, ice and water to the mixture. |
| **3.** | Refrigerate for one hour and then serve fresh. |

**Time: 14 minutes | Serves 2**
Net carbs: 18% (11g/0.4oz) | Fiber: 10% (6g/0.2oz) | Fat: 35% (22g/0.8oz)
Protein: 37% (23g/0.8oz) | Kcal: 345

## Ingredients:

- 2 large eggs
- ¼ cup almond meal
- 2 diced bacon
- 2 tbsp coconut flour
- ½ cup fat-free Greek yogurt
- 2 tsp maple syrup
- 2 tbsp ground flaxseed
- 2 tsp coconut oil
- Ground cinnamon

## Preparation:

| | |
|---|---|
| **1.** | Mix the coconut flour, flaxseed, bacon and almond meal. |
| **2.** | In another bowl, beat the eggs. Then add in the yogurt to create a smooth consistency. |
| **3.** | Stir this into the previously prepared flour mixture. |
| **4.** | Prepare the skillet by heating it up with some oil at medium temperature. |
| **5.** | Drip the pancake batter onto it in four circles. Cook 3 minutes per side. |
| **6.** | Serve the fresh pancakes with maple syrup and cinnamon dust. |

**Time: 11 minutes | Serves 4**

Net carbs: 40% (33g/1.16oz) | Fiber: 13% (11g/0.4oz) | Fat: 16% (13g/0.46oz)
Protein: 28% (23g/0.8oz) | Kcal: 383

## Ingredients:

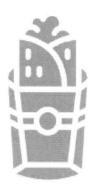

- ◆ 4 egg whites
- ◆ 2 eggs
- ◆ 1 cup shredded Cheddar cheese
- ◆ 4 10-inch whole grain sandwich wraps
- ◆ ½ finely chopped green bell pepper
- ◆ ½ finely chopped red bell pepper
- ◆ ½ finely chopped red onion
- ◆ 1 cup canned black beans
- ◆ 3 tbsp spicy salsa
- ◆ 2 tbsp pickled jalapeno

# Preparation:

| | |
|---|---|
| **1.** | Prepare the sandwich wraps with aluminum foil. Then cook them for a while at medium heat in a toaster oven. |
| **2.** | Beat the eggs and egg whites in a bowl. Then add in the beans. |
| **3.** | Heat up a medium skillet at medium temperature. Then coat it with cooking spray. Cook the egg mixture here for a minute. |
| **4.** | Spread both the bell peppers, jalapeno and cheese on these eggs. Cook this at lowered heat until the cheese has melted. |
| **5.** | Put ¼ of this delicious mixture inside each wrap. Distribute the salsa among these wraps as well. Fold the wraps and serve fresh. |
| **6.** | Refrigerate for one hour and then serve fresh. |

## Time: 10 minutes | Serves 1

Net carbs: 31% (19g/0.7oz) | Fiber: 10% (6g/0.2oz) | Fat: 23% (14g/0.5oz)
Protein: 36% (22g/0.78oz) | Kcal: 310

## Ingredients:

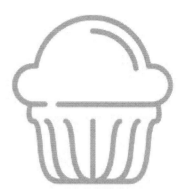

- ♦ 1 large egg
- ♦ ½ cup fat-free Greek yogurt
- ♦ 4 tbsp halved blueberries
- ♦ 2 tbsp almond flour
- ♦ 1 tsp ground flaxseed
- ♦ ½ tsp baking powder
- ♦ 1 tbsp apple sauce
- ♦ 1 tbsp coconut flour
- ♦ 1 tbsp fat-free milk
- ♦ Pinch of salt
- ♦ Pinch of cinnamon

## Preparation:

| | |
|---|---|
| **1.** | Mix both the flours along with baking powder, flaxseed, salt and cinnamon. |
| **2.** | Add whisked eggs to this mixture. Introduce the milk, apple-sauce and half of blueberries to this mouth-watering combination. |
| **3.** | Take a microwave-safe mug and grease it lightly. Pour the mixture into this mug and cook it for about a minute in the oven . |
| **4.** | When the muffin cools down, crumble half of it and fill up the bottom of parfait glass with these crumbles. Spread one layer of yogurt on top. You can make as many layers as you want in this way. |
| **5.** | Finish the topping with the remaining blueberries and serve. |
| **6.** | Serve the fresh pancakes with maple syrup and cinnamon dust. |

**Time: 41 minutes | Serves 4**

Net carbs: 54% (44g/1.55oz) | Fiber: 5% (4g/0.14oz) | Fat: 12% (10g/0.35oz)
Protein: 28% (23g/0.8oz) | Kcal: 373

## Ingredients:

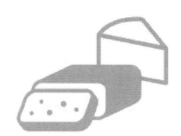

- 8 oz grapefruit juice
- 4 oz cubed whole wheat bread
- 4 oz feta cheese
- 2 ham slices4 egg whites
- 4 eggs
- ½ cup fat-free milk
- 2 sliced tomatoes
- 2 chopped scallions
- 2 cup chopped broccoli florets
- ½cup Greek yogurt
- 3 tbsp ground flaxseed
- 1 1/8 tsp dried oregano

## Preparation:

| | |
|---|---|
| **1.** | Whisk the eggs and egg whites. Then add in the yogurt, milk, flaxseed and oregano. Keep mixing until you reach the expected consistency. |
| **2.** | Then add the broccoli, scallions, ham and bread to this mixture. |
| **3.** | Take a baking dish and spread this mixture. Top it with cheese and tomatoes. |
| **4.** | Bake for roughly 20 minutes. Serve each quarter of this dish with one glass of grapefruit juice. |

## Time: 15 minutes | Serves 1

Net carbs: 38% (23g/0.8oz) | Fiber: 7% (4g/0.14oz) | Fat: 24% (14g/0.5oz)
Protein: 30% (18g/0.6oz) | Kcal: 312

## Ingredients:

- 1 quart water
- 4 0.25-inch thick sweet potato slabs
- 2 tbsp grated cheddar
- 2 large eggs

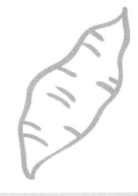

## Preparation:

| | |
|---|---|
| **1.** | Boil the water and then place the eggs inside it using a spoon while lowering the temperature to medium-low. Cook it for 4 minutes covered. |
| **2.** | Drain it later and then place the cooked eggs in cold water. |
| **3.** | Toast the potato slabs at medium-high temperature for 10 minutes. Then cut immediately into half-inch strips. Toss the strips with cheese, salt and pepper. |
| **4.** | Gently put each egg in an egg cup and cut off the top portion. Sprinkle salt and pepper, then dip the potato strips in runny yolks of those eggs. |

**Time: 10 minutes | Serves 1**
Net carbs: 53% (36g/1.27oz) | Fiber: 15% (10g/0.35oz) | Fat: 3% (2g/0.07oz)
Protein: 30% (20g/0.7oz) | Kcal: 345

## Ingredients:

♦ 1 large egg
♦ 1 cup cooked quinoa
♦ ½ cup cannellini beans
♦ ½ cup baby spinach
♦ 1 tbsp water
♦ ½ tsp olive oil
♦ Salt
♦ Pepper

## Preparation:

| 1. | Mix quinoa, beans and spinach in water. Cook this mixture on a non-stick skillet for 2 minutes. |
|---|---|
| 2. | Whisk the egg with pepper and salt. Cook it in olive oil until the yolk reaches your desired state. |
| 3. | Place the quinoa mix on plate and top it with the freshly cooked eggs. |

**Time: 5 minutes | Serves 4**

Net carbs: 74% (20g/0.7oz) | Fiber: 19% (5g/0.18oz) | Fat: 2% (0.5g/0.01oz)

Protein: 4% (1g/0.03oz) | Kcal: 105

## Ingredients:

- 1 thinly sliced apple
- 1 cinnamon stick
- A teapot of boiling water

## Preparation:

| 1. | This is a very simple recipe. Just add the apple slices and cinnamon stick in a teapot of boiling water. Then serve it in four cups with pleasure. |
|----|-----|

**Time: 10 minutes | Serves 1**

Net carbs: 42% (30g/1.1oz) | Fiber: 13% (9g/0.3oz) | Fat: 17% (12g/0.4oz)

Protein: 26% (18g/0.6oz) | Kcal: 330

## Ingredients:

- ¼ cup chopped strawberries
- 1 cup almond milk
- ½ cup rolled oats
- 2 tbsp Greek yogurt
- 2 tbsp peanut butter powder
- 1 tbsp finely chopped peanuts

## Preparation:

| | |
|---|---|
| **1.** | Take a microwave-safe mug. Pour in a mixture of almond milk, peanut butter powder and oats. Stir well so that you are happy with the resulting consistency. |
| **2.** | Cook it in the oven for 3 minutes. |
| **3.** | Add strawberries, peanuts and yogurt before serving. |

### Time: 5 minutes | Serves 4

Net carbs: 60% (12g/0.4oz) | Fiber: 10% (2g/0.07oz) | Fat: 15% (3g/0.1oz)

Protein: 15% (3g/0.1oz) | Kcal: 100

## Ingredients:

- 7 oz chopped pineapple
- 3 oz coconut water
- 1 chopped cucumber
- 1 tsp acai berry powder
- 5 celery sticks

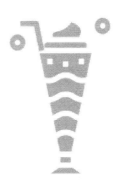

## Preparation:

| 1. | Blend all Ingredients and serve immediately for devouring the fresh fruity flavor. |

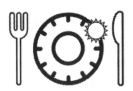

## Time: 24 minutes | Serves 4
Net carbs: 40% (37g/1.3oz) | Fiber: 12% (11g/0.4oz) | Fat: 10% (9g/0.3oz)
Protein: 37% (34g/1.2oz) | Kcal: 40

## Ingredients:

♦ 2 grilled sliced chicken breasts

♦ 1½ lbs asparagus

♦ 2 cups water1 cup green lentils

♦ ½ cup jarred BBQ sauce

♦ ¼ cup toasted and chopped walnuts

♦ 1 chipotle chili

♦ 4 chopped celery stalks

♦ 1 tbsp adobo sauce

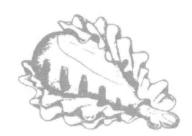

## Preparation:

| 1. | Mix the lentils, chipotle chili and adobo sauce in water. Then transfer this mixture to a rice cooker and cook for 15 minutes. |
|---|---|
| 2. | When the cooker shuts off, add the asparagus immediately and steam until it gets tender. |
| 3. | In another bowl, combine the chicken, walnuts, BBQ sauce and celery. |
| 4. | Transfer the delicious lentil mixture to a bowl. Top it with the BBQ coated chicken and enjoy. |

## Time: 1 hour | Serves 4

Net carbs: % (9g/0.3oz) | Fiber: % (2g/0.07oz) | Fat: % (14g/0.5oz)
Protein: % (26g/0.9oz) | Kcal: 274

## Ingredients:

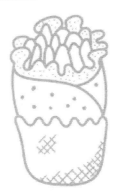

- 1 lb boneless chicken breasts
- 12 lettuce leaves
- 2 garlic cloves
- ½ cup sliced scallions
- 1 sliced cucumber
- ½ cup sliced carrot
- 2 tbsp balsamic vinegar
- 2 tbsp toasted sesame oil
- 2 tbsp thinly sliced fresh ginger
- 2 tbsp toasted sesame seeds
- 2 tbsp reduced-sodium tamari
- 2 tsp sugar
- 2 tsp Chinese chili oil
- 2 tsp ground Sichuan peppercorns

## Preparation:

| | |
|---|---|
| **1.** | Fill up a saucepan with enough water to cover chicken breasts. Then put in the chicken, garlic and ginger. Wait until it reaches the boiling temperature. |
| **2.** | Lower the heat so that it can simmer. When cooked perfectly, transfer it to another plate so that the chicken can cool down. |
| **3.** | Mix the sesame oil, chili oil, vinegar, sugar and peppercorns in another bowl to prepare the sauce. |
| **4.** | Cut the chicken into as many pieces as you want and then toss it with the prepared sauce. |
| **5.** | Serve with lettuce leaves, cucumber, carrots, sesame seeds and scallions as toppings. |

## Time: 25 minutes | Serves 4
Net carbs: 55% (50g/1.76oz) | Fiber: 7% (7g/0.3oz) | Fat: 8% (8g/0.3oz)
Protein: 28% (25g/0.9oz) | Kcal: 400

## Ingredients:

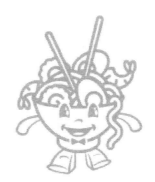

- ½ lbs sliced flank steak
- ½ lbs thinly sliced shiitake
- 6 oz ramen
- ¼ cup chopped cilantro
- 2 cups baby spinach leaves
- 2 cups water
- 2 cups beef broth
- 4 minced garlic cloves
- 4 chopped scallions
- 2 tbsp miso paste
- 2 thinly sliced carrots
- 1 tbsp canola oil

## Preparation:

| | |
|---|---|
| **1.** | Rub the flank steak with miso, cilantro and garlic. |
| **2.** | Heat up a stockpot and add oil to it. Cook the seasoned steak here for a couple of minutes. This will make the outer portion of meat brown but the inner portion will still be pink. |
| **3.** | Transfer the steak to a plate. |
| **4.** | Combine the mushrooms, carrots and scallions. Add this combination to the stockpot and cook at high temperature for 4 minutes. Don't forget to stir from time to time. When the mushroom seems to soften up, add water and broth. |
| **5.** | Add the noodles to this mixture at a lowered temperature. Cover and cook for 2 minutes. |
| **6.** | When the noodles are cooked enough, add spinach to the mix. Then replace the steak and serve after a while. |

**Time: 31 minutes | Serves 4**
Net carbs: 28% (4g/0.14oz) | Fiber: 21% (3g/0.1oz) | Fat: 28% (4g/0.14oz)
Protein: 21% (3g/0.1oz) | Kcal: 67

## Ingredients:

- 1 lb trimmed, sliced asparagus
- 1 bunch of trimmed radishes
- 3 dashes red chili sauce
- 3 cups ice water
- 2 tbsp white vinegar
- 1 tbsp reduced-sodium soy sauce
- 2 tbsp finely chopped scallion
- 2 tsp canola oil
- 1 tsp toasted sesame oil
- ½ tsp grated ginger

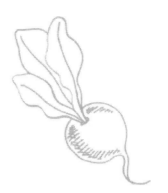

## Preparation:

| | |
|---|---|
| **1.** | Take 1 cup of the ice water in a saucepan with steamer basket and reach a boiling temperature. |
| **2.** | Place the sliced asparagus in the steamer basket of the saucepan. After a minute of steaming, take out the asparagus and place its slices in the rest of ice water. |
| **3.** | Mix the sesame oil, canola oil, chili sauce, soy sauce and vinegar to prepare the dressing. |
| **4.** | Combine asparagus, scallion and radishes in another bowl. Toss this combination with the dressing. Serve fresh and enjoy. |

## Time: 1 hour 5 minutes | Serves 2

Net carbs: 20% (8g/0.3oz) | Fiber: 7% (3g/0.1oz) | Fat: 58% (24g/0.85oz)
Protein: 15% (6g/0.2oz) | Kcal: 100

## Ingredients:

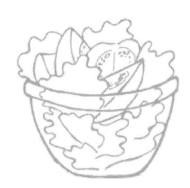

- ◆ 3 sliced radishes
- ◆ 1 sliced broccoli
- ◆ 1 sliced cauliflower
- ◆ 1 tbsp hummus
- ◆ 2 lemon juice
- ◆ 3 oz tomato slices
- ◆ 2 oz sliced onion
- ◆ 1 oz sliced black olives
- ◆ 0.7 oz parsley

## Preparation:

| | |
|---|---|
| **1.** | Blend the cauliflower and broccoli until you are satisfied with the consistency. |
| **2.** | Slowly add the onion and one lemon's juice to this mixture. |
| **3.** | Cook in oven for a minute and refrigerate it for an hour. |
| **4.** | After the mixture is refrigerated enough, add the remaining lemon juice, half of the tomato slices and half of the olives. Blend them well to get the most of each flavor. |
| **5.** | Spread the delicious mixture on a serving plate. Sprinkle the remaining portion of olives, tomatoes and onions on it. |
| **6.** | Serve with hummus. |

## Time: 1 hour | Serves 4

Net carbs: % (20g/0.7oz) | Fiber: % (5g/0.18oz) | Fat: % (11g/0.4oz)
Protein: % (32g/1.2oz) | Kcal: 400

## Ingredients:

- 2 lbs baking potatoes
- ¼ lb lean ground turkey
- 4 oz chopped turkey bacon
- ⅓ cup sour cream
- 4 thinly sliced scallions
- 2 cups thinly sliced baby spinach
- ½ cup crumbled feta cheese
- 8 cups shredded lettuce
- 1 tsp hot sauce
- ½ cup fat-free Greek yogurt
- 2 tbsp dried onion
- 1 tbsp olive oil
- ½ tsp garlic powder
- Water

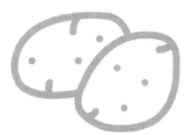

## Preparation:

| | |
|---|---|
| **1.** | Fill up ¼ of a large stockpot with water. When it boils, leave the potatoes in the water and cook them this way until it gets tender. |
| **2.** | Cut these boiled potatoes in half. Scoop out the central portion. Preserve these fillings in a separate bowl. |
| **3.** | Combine the fillings with spinach, sour cream, hot sauce and yogurt. Make sure the consistency is smooth enough. |
| **4.** | Preheat the oven to 390-degrees Fahrenheit. |
| **5.** | Heat up oil in a skillet. Cook the potato skins for 2 minutes until they turn brown. Place these cooked skins on a baking sheet. |
| **6.** | Combine turkey, bacon, dried onion and garlic powder. Add this mixture to the previous skillet. Cook them until the pink hue leaves the meat. |
| **7.** | Fill up the empty side of each potato skin with this turkey mixture. Add a layer of the potato mixture on it. Sprinkle the scallions and cheese over it. Bake this delicious setup for 15 minutes. |
| **8.** | Serve immediately with lettuce. |

## Time: 1 hour 20 minutes | Serves1

Net carbs: 57% (50g/1.76oz) | Fiber: 17% (15g/0.5oz) | Fat: 10% (9g/0.3oz)
Protein: 16% (14g/0.5oz) | Kcal: 380

## Ingredients:

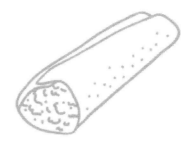

- ◆ 8 corn tortillas
- ◆ 8 oz tomatillos
- ◆ 4 cups diced butternut squash
- ◆ 2 cups cooked pinto beans
- ◆ ⅔ cup cilantro
- ◆ ½cup finely chopped green cabbage
- ◆ ¼ cup sliced white onion
- ◆ 4 finely chopped garlic cloves
- ◆ 3 small snipped dried red chilies
- ◆ 1 jalapeno pepper
- ◆ ½ diced avocado
- ◆ 8 tsp feta cheese
- ◆ 1 tsp salt
- ◆ ¾ tsp dried and divided oregano
- ◆ ½ tsp chili powder
- ◆ ¼ tsp cumin seeds
- ◆ Pepper
- ◆ Water

## Preparation:

| | |
|---|---|
| **1.** | Get rid of the husks on tomatillos. After a thorough rinse, cook them in boiling water for 5 minutes. Then drain the cooked tomatillos and place on a plate. |
| **2.** | Take a skillet and heat it up at medium temperature. Then toast the onions, jalapenos and garlic cloves there for 5 minutes. |
| **3.** | After they cools down, peel cut off the stems and seeds of jalapeno. Then blend these jalapenos, half of garlic, tomatillos, onions and avocado with a food processor. Keep doing so until the mixture turns smooth in consistency. |
| **4.** | Add in salt, pepper and cilantro in the end. Place it by the side to serve as the taco topping. |
| **5.** | Combine squash, chilis, garlic, half of the salt, ½ tsp oregano, oil and cumin seeds. Then spread this mixture on a baking sheet and bake for about half an hour. |
| **6.** | When it cools down, stir in the remaining garlic pieces into the mixture. |
| **7.** | In another bowl, season the beans with ground cumin, pepper, chili powder, rest of the oregano and salt. Cook this concoction for 10 minutes in a saucepan at medium-low temperature. |
| **8.** | Warm up the tortillas one by one in a skillet to make them soft enough for serving. Then fill each with a quarter of the bean mixture and some of the roasted squash. Top them with cabbage, cilantro, salsa and cheese while serving. |

## Time: 40 minutes | Serves 4

Net carbs: 48% (23g/0.8oz) | Fiber: 23% (11g/0.4oz) | Fat: 8% (4g/0.14oz)
Protein: 20% (10g/0.35oz) | Kcal: 200

## Ingredients:

- 2 15-oz cans of black beans
- 3 cups water
- ½ cup salsa
- 1 tbsp lime juice
- 1 chopped onion
- 1 tbsp canola oil
- 4 tbsp sour cream
- 2 tbsp chopped cilantro
- 1 tbsp chili powder
- ¼ tsp salt
- 1 tsp ground cumin

## Preparation:

| | |
|---|---|
| **1.** | Cook the onions in a saucepan until they get soft in texture. |
| **2.** | Add cumin and chili powder to create the mouth-watering flavor. Stir for a minute. |
| **3.** | Then add salsa, salt and beans with more water to the concoction. When it reaches the boiling temperature, reduce the heat and let it simmer for a while. |
| **4.** | Take it out from the stove and then add some lime juice into the mix. |
| **5.** | Pour half of the soup into a blender and start the machine. Add the resulting puree to the saucepan. |
| **6.** | Serve the dish with cilantro and sour cream. |

## Time: 50 minutes | Serves4
Net carbs: 50% (43g/1.5oz) | Fiber: 20% (17g/0.6oz) | Fat: 10% (9g/0.3oz)
Protein: 20% (17g/0.6oz) | Kcal: 354

## Ingredients:

- 1 15-oz can of black beans
- 1 16-inch long baguette
- 1 tbsp chopped pickled jalapeno
- 1 pitted ripe avocado
- 1½ cups shredded green cabbage
- 3 tbsp salsa
- 2 tbsp minced onion
- 1 tbsp lime juice
- ½ tsp ground cumin

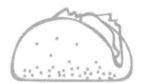

## Preparation:

| | |
|---|---|
| **1.** | Mix beans, jalapeno, salsa and cumin well. |
| **2.** | Combine avocado and onion. Mash them together with the help of some lime juice. |
| **3.** | Make four equal pieces out of the baguette. Then cut each of those in half. Now scoop out the soft bread part in its central portion. This will leave you with the crust portion mostly. |
| **4.** | Spread the bean paste, cabbage and avocado mixture into each of these pieces as filling. Serve immediately. |

**Time: 50 minutes | Serves 4**

Net carbs: 26% (6g/0.2oz) | Fiber: 9% (2g/0.07oz) | Fat: 40% (9g/0.3oz)

Protein: 26% (6g/0.2oz) | Kcal: 127

## Ingredients:

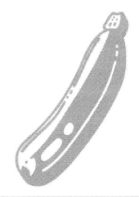

- 1 lb sliced zucchini
- 1 chopped medium onion
- 1 4-oz can diced green chilis
- ½ cup grated cheddar cheese
- 1 tbsp canola oil
- ¼ tsp salt

## Preparation:

| | |
|---|---|
| **1.** | On a hot non-stick skillet or pan of oil, stir in onion and zucchini with the lids covered. When they start turning light brown, add in the salt and chili. |
| **2.** | Take out this combination in a bowl so that you can mash it well. When its consistency gets smooth and chunky, introduce the cheese into the delicious mixture. |

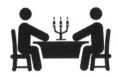

**Time: 2 hours 31 minutes | Serves 4**
Net carbs: 33% (12g/0.4oz) | Fiber: 3% (1g/0.03oz) | Fat: 5% (2g/0.07oz)
Protein: 58% (21g/0.74oz) | Kcal: 150

## Ingredients:

- 1 turkey breast tenderloin
- 8 8-inch skewers
- ½ cup coconut water
- ¼ cup lime juice
- ½ cup flaked and toasted coconut
- 2 tbsp honey
- ½ tsp shredded lime peel
- ¼ tsp crushed red pepper

## Preparation:

| | |
|---|---|
| **1.** | Take water, lime juice, honey, lime peel and red pepper in a large plastic bag. This combination will serve as the marinade. |
| **2.** | Cut out the turkey to carve thin strips out of it. Add this to the marinade and seal the bag. Then shake it a little to coat the meat properly. Refrigerate it for 3 hours. |
| **3.** | After refrigerating, get rid of the marinade liquid and drain the meat. Place the turkey on the skewers and grill them under cover for 8 minutes. You should turn it over once halfway. |
| **4.** | Spread some coconut flakes over the skewers while serving. |

## Time: 1 hour 24 minutes | Serves 6

Net carbs: 8% (3g/0.1oz) | Fiber: 3% (1g/0.03oz) | Fat: 20% (8g/0.3oz)
Protein: 68% (25g/0.9oz) | Kcal: 190

## Ingredients:

- 6 chicken breast fillets
- 2 cups almond milk
- ¾ cup chopped green chili
- ½ cup chicken broth
- 3 sliced scallions
- 1 thinly sliced garlic clove
- 3 tbsp toasted almonds
- 2 tbsp whipping cream
- 1 tbsp canola oil
- 1 tbsp toasted sesame seeds
- ¾ tsp salt

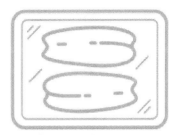

## Preparation:

| | |
|---|---|
| **1.** | Mix in almond milk, almonds, chicken broth, chili, scallions, garlic and half the salt. Cook this combination until the temperature reaches a boiling point. Reduce the heat and let it simmer until the quantity becomes half. |
| **2.** | Blend the mixture to prepare a smooth puree which will function as the sauce. |
| **3.** | Spread the rest of salt on the chicken. Then cook it with oil on a non-stick skillet until they turn brown. You can do so in batches. |
| **4.** | Return the cooked chicken into pan and add the sauce. Simmer at a lower temperature and cook for 5 minutes. You can stir in the cream as well. |
| **5.** | Serve the delicious chicken dish with scallion greens and sesame seeds. |

**Time: 1 hour | Serves 8**

Net carbs: 45% (30g/1.1oz) | Fiber: 9% (6g/0.2oz) | Fat: 9% (6g/0.2oz)
Protein: 36% (24g/0.85oz) | Kcal: 290

## Ingredients:

- 1 lb cooked and diced shrimp
- 1 15-oz can of refried beans
- 2 4-oz cans of chopped green chili
- 12 corn tortillas
- 1 lime
- 2 cups green salsa
- 1 cup shredded cheese
- 1 cup thawed corn
- ½ cup chopped cilantro

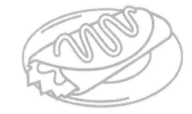

## Preparation:

| | |
|---|---|
| **1.** | Preheat the oven to 425-degrees in Fahrenheit. Prepare the baking dish by coating with some cooking spray. |
| **2.** | Take a microwave-safe bowl. Combine the shrimp, corn, one quarter of salsa and chili in it. Bake this combination for a couple of minutes. |
| **3.** | Spread another quarter of the salsa on the baking dish. Arrange half of the tortillas on it in one layer. Top this layer with refried beans and shrimp mixture respectively. Cover them with the remaining tortillas. Pour in the remaining salsa over it. |
| **4.** | Bake it for 20 minutes covered in foil. After that, spread the cheese on top and bake for a little longer. When the cheese melts completely, serve with lime and cilantro. |

**Time: 50 minutes | Serves 4**
Net carbs: 30% (23g/0.8oz) | Fiber: 8% (6g/0.2oz) | Fat: 15% (12g/0.4oz)
Protein: 47% (36g/1.27oz) | Kcal: 380

## Ingredients:

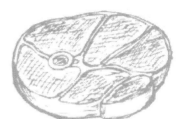

- 1 jar taco sauce
- ¼ cup water
- ¼ tsp cayenne pepper
- 1 lb lean ground beef
- 1 tbsp chili powder
- 1 can kidney beans
- 1 chopped red bell pepper
- 6 chopped garlic cloves
- 1 chopped large onion
- 1⅔ tsp ground cumin

## Preparation:

| | |
|---|---|
| **1.** | Firstly, cook the beef with onion and bell pepper at medium temperature. During the process, break down the meat with a spoon. Stop when it turns brownish. |
| **2.** | Add garlic, cumin, cayenne and chili powder for instilling a beautiful fragrance into the dish. |
| **3.** | Stir in taco sauce and water before letting it simmer. |
| **4.** | When the vegetables reach a tender texture, add beans and cook for one more minute. |

## Time: 1 hour 5 minutes | Serves 4

Net carbs: 45% (32g/1.13oz) | Fiber: 7% (5g/0.18oz) | Fat: 8% (6g/0.2oz)
Protein: 39% (27g/0.95oz) | Kcal: 300

## Ingredients:

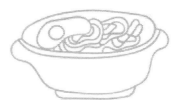

- 12 oz pork tenderloin
- 4 oz buckwheat noodles or soba
- 4 sliced medium carrots
- 1 thinly sliced stalk celery
- 3 cups water
- 3 cups sliced trimmed bok choy
- 2 cups trimmed snow peas
- 2 cups thinly sliced button mushrooms
- 1 tbsp soy sauce
- ½cup thinly sliced green onions
- 1 cup unsalted chicken broth
- 4 tbsp orange juice
- 1 tbsp canola oil
- 1 tbsp flour
- ¼ tsp ground ginger
- 1 tsp five-spice powder

## Preparation:

| | |
|---|---|
| **1.** | Add ginger and five-spice powder to the pork strips. |
| **2.** | Coat a nonstick oven with some cooking spray and warm it up at a medium-high temperature. Cook the seasoned pork strips here for 5 minutes. |
| **3.** | After removing the cooked pork from it, add carrots, celery and mushroom to the pot. Cook this mixture for a few minutes at medium heat. Add broth and water before reaching the boiling temperature. |
| **4.** | Add soba to this mixture and keep on cooking until the noodles become soft enough. |
| **5.** | In a separate bowl, combine soy sauce and flour to reach a smooth consistency. Add this combination, bok choy, onions, snow peas and the cooked pork to noodles. Keep cooking until it reaches the boiling temperature. |
| **6.** | Before serving, add in the orange juice. |

## Time: 1 hour 21 minutes | Serves 8

Net carbs: 43% (35g/1.23oz) | Fiber: 5% (4g/0.14oz) | Fat: 20% (17g/0.6oz)
Protein: 32% (26g/0.9oz) | Kcal: 410

## Ingredients:

- 14 oz coconut milk
- 1 lb boneless chicken breast
- 14 oz tofu
- 14 oz diced tomatoes
- 1 tsp ground turmeric
- 8 oz cooked bean thread noodles
- 6 thinly sliced scallions
- 1 tbsp ground coriander
- 2 diced and seeded chili
- 3 sliced hard-boiled eggs
- 1 tsp curry powder
- 1 chopped ginger
- 5½ cups chicken broth
- ½ cup chopped cilantro
- 3 cups mung bean sprouts
- 2 cups sliced onions
- ¼ cup macadamia nuts
- 2 tbsp soy sauce
- 3 tbsp fish sauce
- 2 tbsp peanut oil
- 2 tsp brown sugar
- 2 tbsp lime juice
- 2 tsp ground cumin
- 1 tsp ground fennel seed

## Preparation:

| | |
|---|---|
| **1.** | Blend the combination of onions, nuts, coriander, fish sauce, curry powder, brown sugar, coriander, turmeric, cumin, garlic, ginger, pepper and fennel. Make a smooth paste out of this combination. |
| **2.** | Cook this delicious mixture in hot oil for 5 minutes. Then introduce the chicken broth and let it simmer for about 10 minutes. |
| **3.** | Add lime juice, coconut milk and soy sauce to it. Let it simmer again for a while. |
| **4.** | Cut the chicken breasts into bite-sized pieces or shred them. |
| **5.** | Add tomatoes, bean sprouts and tofu to the soup. Cook for a couple of minutes before adding the shredded chicken. |
| **6.** | While serving, first arrange the cooked noodles in 8 bowls. Then pour in the soup over each. Top each noodles-soup bowl with egg slices, cilantro and scallions. |

**Time: 44 minutes | Serves 4**

Net carbs: 31% (16g/0.6oz) | Fiber: 10% (5g/0.18oz) | Fat: 15% (8g/0.3oz)

Protein: 43% (22g/0.78oz) | Kcal: 240

## Ingredients:

- 1 lb mackerel, cut into 4 pieces
- 8 oz trimmed okra
- 2 sliced tomatoes
- 2 tbsp chopped ginger
- 2 tsp ground cumin
- 2 halved serrano chili
- 3 chopped garlic cloves
- 2 cups water
- 1 tsp brown sugar
- ¾ cup sliced shallots
- 2 tbsp peanut oil
- 1⅔ tbsp tamarind paste
- 1 tbsp ground coriander
- 1 tbsp chili powder
- 2 tsp ground turmeric
- ½ tsp mustard seeds
- 1 tsp salt

## Preparation:

| | |
|---|---|
| **1.** | Warm up a skillet by heating the peanut oil at medium temperature. Cook garlic, ginger, mustard seeds and shallots in it for 5 minutes. |
| **2.** | Now add coriander, chili powder, turmeric and cumin to the concoction. Stir them until you can sense the spicy fragrance. |
| **3.** | Mix the tamarind and water in another bowl. Now add this mixture to the cooking dish, along with chili, okra, salt and brown sugar. Put the lid on and let it cook for 7 minutes. |
| **4.** | Stir in tomatoes and fish so that its pieces are covered by the spicy liquid. Let it simmer for 5 minutes. Serve when it has cooled down. |

## Time: 1 hour 31 minutes | Serves 6

Net carbs: 21% (9g/0.3oz) | Fiber: 2% (1g/0.03oz) | Fat: 10% (4g/0.14oz)

Protein: 66% (28g/1oz) | Kcal: 180

## Ingredients:

- ◆ 8 oz ground turkey
- ◆ 1 lightly beaten egg
- ◆ ¾ cup finely chopped sweet pepper
- ◆ 1 seeded chopped jalapeno chili pepper
- ◆ ☐ cup yellow cornmeal
- ◆ ½ cup taco sauce
- ◆ ½ cup thinly sliced green onions
- ◆ ¼ cup fat-free milk
- ◆ ¼ tsp salt
- ◆ 1 tbsp taco seasoning

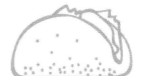

## Preparation:

| | |
|---|---|
| **1.** | Get the oven ready by preheating it to 350-degrees Fahrenheit. |
| **2.** | Whisk milk and egg in a bowl. Slowly stir in taco seasoning, cornmeal, salt, jalapeno pepper, sweet pepper, onion and turkey. Place this mixture on a loaf pan and bake for 44 minutes. |
| **3.** | Pour in taco sauce on top of the meatloaf and bake again for 8 minutes. |
| **4.** | Cut the loaf into 12 pieces and serve 2 slices on each plate. |

**Time:1 hour 43 minutes | Serves 8**
Net carbs: 31% (20g/0.7oz) | Fiber: 5% (3g/0.1oz) | Fat: 28% (18g/0.6oz)
Protein: 36% (23g/0.8oz) | Kcal: 340

## Ingredients:

- 16 poblano peppers
- 6 large egg whites
- 1 bunch of chopped scallions
- 2 cups shredded cooked chicken
- 2 cups thawed corn
- 2 cups shredded Mexican cheese
- □ cup all-purpose flour
- ½ cup non-fat yogurt
- 1½ tsp salt
- 4 tbsp canola oil

## Preparation:

| | |
|---|---|
| **1.** | Broil the peppers for 10 minutes until its skin turns blackened. |
| **2.** | When they cool down, take out the blistered skin and obtain the whole stems. Cut each in half, deseed and put aside. |
| **3.** | In a separate bowl, mix chicken, cheese, yogurt, scallions and 1 tsp salt. Now feel the peppers with a quarter of this mixture. |
| **4.** | Mix the rest of the salt with flour so that the peppers can be dipped into it. Similarly, whisk the egg whites in another plate for dipping. Then coat each pepper with the flour dip and the egg whites respectively. |
| **5.** | Cook the peppers in hot oil until the cheese melts. |

**Time: 30 minutes | Serves 4**
Net carbs: 28% (16g/0.6oz) | Fiber: 3% (2g/0.07oz) | Fat: 21% (12g/0.4oz)
Protein: 47% (27g/0.95oz) | Kcal: 280

## Ingredients:

- 1 lb salmon fillet
- 2 dried red chilis
- 4 minced garlic cloves
- 1 cup diced ripe mango
- ½ cup sliced shallot
- 3 tsp extra-virgin olive oil
- 2 tbsp chopped cilantro
- 2 tsp coriander seed
- ½ tsp salt

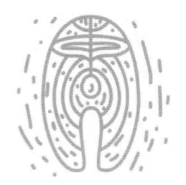

## Preparation:

| | |
|---|---|
| **1.** | Cook shallot, chilis and coriander in 1 tsp oil for a couple of minutes. Now blend this mixture with mango and remaining oil to prepare the sauce. |
| **2.** | Mix garlic and salt to use as seasoning for salmon. Then broil the fillet until its center turns opaque. |
| **3.** | Serve the cooked fillet with hot sauce and cilantro. |

**Time: 2 hours 22 minutes | Serves6**

Net carbs: 88% (52g/1.83oz) | Fiber: 7% (4g/0.14oz) | Fat: 2% (1g/0.03oz)

Protein: 2% (1g/0.03oz) | Kcal: 190

## Ingredients:

- 6 cups frozen mixed berries
- 1 cup basil
- 1 cup sugar
- 1 cup water
- ¾ cup lemon juice

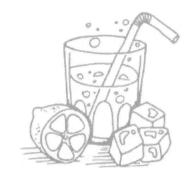

## Preparation:

| | |
|---|---|
| **1.** | Mix sugar and water to cook at high temperature. |
| **2.** | Add basil and turn off the heat. Let it cool down. |
| **3.** | Strain the resulting syrup in another bowl and freeze it. |
| **4.** | Blend the berries and lemon juice with this syrup. |
| **5.** | Spread the puree on a baking tray covered with plastic wrap. Refrigerate it for 2 hours. |

## Time: 45 minutes | Serves 6

Net carbs: 40% (30g/1.1oz) | Fiber: 7% (5g/0.18oz) | Fat: 22% (17g/0.6oz)
Protein: 30% (23g/0.8oz) | Kcal: 400

## Ingredients:

- ◆  1 lb lean ground beef
- ◆  2 minced garlic cloves
- ◆  6 whole-wheat tortillas
- ◆  1 can chopped green chilis
- ◆  1 cup chopped onion
- ◆  1½ cups shredded lettuce
- ◆  1 cup finely chopped mushrooms
- ◆  1 cup canned refried beans
- ◆  6 tbsp shredded cheddar cheese
- ◆  1 tbsp extra-virgin olive oil
- ◆  6 tbsp tomato salsa
- ◆  1 tbsp chili powder
- ◆  1 tsp ground cumin
- ◆  1 tsp dried oregano
- ◆  ½ tsp kosher salt
- ◆  Olive oil cooking spray

## Preparation:

| | |
|---|---|
| **1.** | Cook garlic and onion in hot oil for 2 minutes. |
| **2.** | Add beef, cumin, chili powder, oregano, mushrooms and salt to it. Then cook again until the pink color leaves beef. |
| **3.** | Slowly stir in the chilies and refried beans. Cook for 2 more minutes. |
| **4.** | Coat a baking sheet with some cooking spray. Fill up each tortilla with as much of the beef mix as you want. Top them with some cheese and wrap each up like a burrito. |
| **5.** | Bake them for 15 minutes. Serve with salsa and lettuce. |

## Time: 1 hour 25 minutes | Serves 4
Net carbs: 60% (30g/1.1oz) | Fiber: 4% (3g/0.1oz) | Fat: 1% (1g/0.03oz)
Protein: 30% (15g/0.5oz) | Kcal: 190

## Ingredients:

- ◆ 1 lb dry sea scallops
- ◆ 2 chopped ripe mangoes
- ◆ ☐ cup lemon juice
- ◆ ¾ cup sliced chili peppers
- ◆ ☐ cup sliced onion
- ◆ ¾ tsp salt

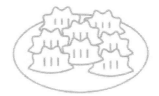

## Preparation:

| | |
|---|---|
| 1. | Cook the scallops in simmering water until they are firm enough. After they are cooked, transfer them to a bowl. |
| 2. | Add half of the mango to the scallops. Puree the other half with lemon juice and salt. |
| 3. | Now add the puree on the scallops. Toss it with onion and chili peppers. |
| 4. | Refrigerate it for about an hour and serve fresh. |

## Time: 40 minutes | Serves 8

Net carbs: 60% (22g/0.78z) | Fiber: 11% (4g/0.14oz) | Fat: 16% (6g/0.2oz)
Protein: 14% (5g/0.18oz) | Kcal: 165

## Ingredients:

♦ 2 peeled and diced apples

♦ 4 dates

♦ □ cup fat-free cream cheese

♦ ½ cup walnut halves

♦ □ cup fat-free Greek yogurt

♦ 3 tbsp coconut sugar

♦ ¼ tsp cinnamon

♦ Pinch of sea salt

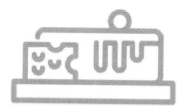

## Preparation:

| | |
|---|---|
| **1.** | Combine cinnamon, salt and □ of the coconut sugar with apples. Cook it at medium heat until the apples are boiled. Then lower the heat and simmer for half an hour. Let it cool down. |
| **2.** | Mix cheese, yogurt and the rest of coconut sugar in a separate bowl. Beat this mixture until the sugar dissolves. Then store it in the refrigerator until it has settled down. |
| **3.** | Blend dates and walnuts to create a crumb-like consistency. |
| **4.** | Then layer the walnut mixture, cream cheese and cooked apples in each dessert dish. Refrigerate before serving. |

**Time: 50 minutes | Serves 4**

Net carbs: 20% (12g/0.4oz) | Fiber: 10% (5g/0.18oz) | Fat: 40% (27g/0.95oz)

Protein: 14% (7g/0.3oz) | Kcal: 242

## Ingredients:

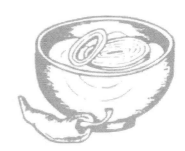

- ◆ 2 seeded and diced red bell peppers
- ◆ 2 chopped green chilis
- ◆ 1 diced onion
- ◆ 2 cups vegetable broth
- ◆ ½ cup unsalted shelled pistachios
- ◆ ¼ cup chopped cilantro
- ◆ 2 tbsp canola oil
- ◆ 2 tbsp whipping cream
- ◆ 1 cup nonfat buttermilk
- ◆ 2 tsp sweet paprika
- ◆ 1 tsp sea salt
- ◆ ½ tsp ground cardamom

PEPPER AND PAPRIKA SOUP

**65**

## Preparation:

| | |
|---|---|
| **1.** | Cook the combination of bell peppers, onion and chili at medium-high temperature for 5 minutes. |
| **2.** | Add salt, cardamom and paprika to the mix for a couple of minutes. |
| **3.** | Stir in pistachios and broth. Keep cooking until it reaches a boiling temperature. Then lower the heat and simmer for about half an hour. |
| **4.** | When it cools down, blend this soup to prepare a smooth puree. Then put it back into the cooking pan. |
| **5.** | In a separate bowl, beat cream and buttermilk together. Add this into the soup slowly. |
| **6.** | Serve the soup with some cilantro on top. |

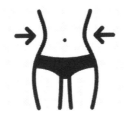

Metabolism reset diet aims at increasing your metabolic rate through the right dietary habits and drastic lifestyle changes. If you don't know where to begin, let us help by introducing our 30-day weight loss plan tailored to attain metabolism rest goals. Every single day, we have introduced a new recipe meal to keep it exciting and full of food adventures. You can invest in the following metabolism reset diet plan to reduce your weight.

*Breakfast:* **Blueberry French Toast**

### Serves 4/25 min

Net carbs: 64% (55g/1.94oz) | Fiber: 8% (7g/0.3oz) | Fat: 8% (7g/0.3oz) | Protein: 20% (17g/0.6oz) | kcal: 390

## Ingredients:

- 8 whole-wheat bread slices
- 2 cup blueberries
- 2 large egg whites
- 1 cup fat-free milk
- 1 large egg

- ½ cup cottage cheese
- ⅓ cup sugar
- 1 tbsp canola oil
- 1 tsp vanilla extract

## Preparation:

| 1. | Blend the blueberries, cottage cheese, sugar and half of the milk. |
|----|----|
| 2. | In another bowl, whisk the eggs, egg whites, vanilla extract and remaining milk. |
| 3. | Spread the blueberry mix between each pair of bread slices. |
| 4. | Heat up the skillet with ½ tbsp oil and cook the stuffed breads for a couple of minutes per side. |
| 5. | Serve fresh and warm. |

*Lunch:* **BBQ Chicken Salad**

*Dinner:* **Turkey Skewers with Coconut**

*Breakfast:* **Berry Blast**

*Lunch:* **Chicken and Mango Salad**

### Serves 4/20 min

Net carbs: 32% (20g/0.7oz) | Fiber: 8% (5g/0.18oz) | Fat: 14% (9g/0.3oz) | Protein: 44% (27g/0.95oz) | kcal: 285

## Ingredients:

- 1 sliced mango
- 6 cups sliced napa cabbage
- 2 cups cooked and shredded chicken breast
- 2 cups sliced sugar snap peas
- ½ cup chopped mint

- ⅓ cup orange juice
- 3 tbsp rice vinegar
- ¼ cup sliced scallions
- 3 tbsp soy sauce
- 2 tbsp toasted sesame seeds
- 1 tbsp toasted sesame oil

## Preparation:

| | |
|---|---|
| **1.** | Whisk soy sauce, vinegar, juice and sesame oil. |
| **2.** | Add chicken, cabbage, mango, peas, mint and scallions. |
| **3.** | Serve with some sprinkles of sesame seeds. |

*Dinner:* **Chicken Breasts with Almond Cream Sauce**

*Breakfast:* **Almond and Bacon Pancakes**

*Lunch:* **Chicken Lettuce Wraps**

*Dinner:* **Black Bean Burgers**

### Serves 8/30 min

Net carbs: 48% (40g/1.41oz) | Fiber: 14% (11g/0.4oz) | Fat: 22% (18g/0.6oz) | Protein: 15% (12g/0.4oz) | kcal: 400

## Ingredients:

- 8 toasted whole-grain burger buns
- 8 tomato slices
- 2 cans of black beans, mashed
- 1 large beaten egg
- 1 cup tortilla chips
- 1 cup sprouts
- ½ cup drained salsa

- ½ cup guacamole
- ½ cup grated onion
- 3 tbsp mayonnaise
- 3 tbsp avocado oil
- 4 tsp chili powder
- 2 tsp ground cumin
- 1 tsp salt

## Preparation:

| | |
|---|---|
| **1.** | Combine the mashed black beans, salsa, egg, mayonnaise, onion, tortilla chips, cumin, chili powder and salt. |
| **2.** | Pour ⅓ cup of this mixture into each burger. |
| **3.** | Cook the four burgers in a non-stick skillet until they are brown. |
| **4.** | Serve with guacamole, sprouts and tomato slices. |

*Breakfast:* **Cookie Crunch Smoothie**

### Serves 1/10 min

Net carbs: 63% (55g/1.94oz) | Fiber: 10% (9g/0.3oz) | Fat: 13% (11g/0.4oz) | Protein: 14% (12g/0.4oz) | Kcal: 390

## Ingredients:

- 3 chocolate cookie wafers
- 4 ice cubes
- 1 cup fat-free milk
- 2 tbsp ground flaxseed
- 2 tsp sugar
- ½ tsp vanilla extract

## Preparation:

| **1.** | Blend all the Ingredients and serve fresh! |

*Lunch:* **Miso Beef Ramen**

*Dinner:* **Baked Shrimp Enchilada**

*Breakfast:* **Breakfast Burrito**

*Lunch:* **Chicken and Kale Salad with Avocado Ranch**

### Serves 4/26 min

Net carbs: 25% (20g/0.7oz) | Fiber: 10% (8g/0.3oz) | Fat: 24% (23g/0.8oz) | Protein: 37% (30g/1.1oz) | kcal: 420

## Ingredients:

- 1 ripe avocado
- 8 cups shredded kale
- 2 cups shredded cooked chicken breast
- 1½ cups tortilla chips
- 1 cup rinsed black beans
- ½ cup chopped mango
- ⅓ cup ranch dressing
- ¼ cup diced onion
- ¼ cup shredded cheddar cheese
- 2 tbsp chopped pickled jalapenos
- 1 tbsp white wine vinegar
- ¼ tsp ground pepper
- Crushed red pepper
- Lime wedges

## Preparation:

| 1. | Blend the jalapenos, avocado, ranch dressing, pepper and vinegar to create a smooth puree. |
|---|---|
| 2. | Mix this puree with chicken, kale, beans, mango, tortilla chips, onion and cheese. |
| 3. | Serve with red pepper and lime wedges. |

*Dinner:* **Beef Bean Verde**

*Breakfast:* **Blueberry Muffin Parfait**

*Lunch:* **Radish and Asparagus Salad**

*Dinner:* **Mini Chili Casseroles**

### Serves 8/40 min

Net carbs: 35% (12g/0.4oz) | Fiber: 6% (2g/0.07oz) | Fat: 21% (7g/0.3oz) | Protein: 70% (23g/0.8oz) | kcal: 200

## Ingredients:

- 8-oz diced green chilis
- 4 large eggs
- 6 large egg whites
- 4 sliced scallions
- 1 cup shredded cheddar cheese
- 1½ cup nonfat milk
- ¾ cup corn
- ¼ tsp salt

## Preparation:

| | |
|---|---|
| **1.** | Mix eggs, egg whites, milk and salt. |
| **2.** | Distribute the egg mixture, corn, scallions, and chilis among ramekins evenly with cheese toppings. |
| **3.** | Bake them for about half an hour. |

*Breakfast:* **Frittata Muffins**

### Serves 4/27 min

Net carbs: 12% (7g/0.3oz) | Fiber: 3% (2g/0.07oz) | Fat: 43% (25g/0.9oz) | Protein: 40% (23g/0.8oz) | kcal: 350

## Ingredients:

- 4 large eggs
- 2 diced bacon
- 1 tbsp milk
- 2 cups chopped kale
- ¼ sliced red onion
- 1 tbsp olive oil
- ⅛ tsp black pepper
- ⅛ tsp kosher salt

## Preparation:

| 1. | Cook onion, bacon and spinach on a skillet till the onion gets tender. Set them in a muffin pan. |
| 2. | In another bowl, combine milk, eggs, salt and pepper. Pour this over the layer of vegetables in the muffin pan. Bake for 10 minutes. |

*Lunch:* **Veggie Tabbouleh**

*Dinner:* **Pork and Soba Noodles**

*Breakfast:* **Boiled Eggs and Sweet Potatoes**

*Lunch:* **Chipotle Beef-Potato Salad**

### Serves 6/1 hour 30 min

Net carbs: 24% (10g/0.35oz) | Fiber: 10% (4g/0.14oz) | Fat: 34% (14g/0.5oz) | Protein: 32% (13g/0.46oz) | kcal: 240

## Ingredients:

- 1 quart water
- 12 oz diced stew beef
- 3 boiled potatoes
- 2 chopped garlic cloves
- 1 diced onion
- 1 diced ripe avocado
- 3 tbsp cider vinegar
- 2 tbsp chopped chipotle chili
- 1 tsp salt

## Preparation:

| | |
|---|---|
| **1.** | When the water starts to boil, add beef, salt and garlic to it. |
| **2.** | When it starts to boil again, lower the heat and let it simmer for an hour. |
| **3.** | Transfer the meat to a plate for cooling down. Then shred it accordingly. |
| **4.** | Use the meat broth to simmer the potatoes for 15 minutes. |
| **5.** | Then sprinkle the cooked potatoes with some vinegar. |
| **6.** | Mix the shredded beef with the potatoes, onion, chipotle and oil. |
| **7.** | When it cools down, serve with avocado. |

*Dinner:* **Chicken Noodle Soup**

*Breakfast:* **Quinoa Porridge**

*Lunch:* **Bean Tacos with Green Salsa**

*Dinner:* **Summer Squash Casserole**

### Serves 12/1 hour 25 min

Net carbs: 30% (7g/0.3oz) | Fiber: 8% (2g/0.07oz) | Fat: 30% (7g/0.3oz) | Protein: 30% (7g/0.3oz) | kcal: 125

## Ingredients:

- 4.5 oz chopped jalapenos
- 4 oz chopped chilis
- 4 thinly sliced scallions
- 10 cups quartered summer squash
- 2 cups grated cheddar cheese

- ¾ cup mild salsa
- ⅔ cup chopped yellow onion
- ¼ cup chopped red onion
- ¼ cup all-purpose flour
- ½ tsp salt

## Preparation:

| | |
|---|---|
| **1.** | Mix the squash, chilis, jalapenos, salt, onion and half of the cheese. Add in flour and toss for coating. Bake this mixture to form the casserole for 45 minutes. |
| **2.** | Spread salsa and rest of cheese on the baked casserole. Return it to the oven to bake for 30 more minutes. |
| **3.** | Sprinkle scallions on top before serving. |

*Breakfast:* **Baked Tomato Cups with Egg and Bacon**

### Serves 1/15 min

Net carbs: 8% (4g/0.14oz) | Fiber: 2% (1g/0.03oz) | Fat: 32% (16g/0.6oz) | Protein: 58% (29g/1oz) | kcal: 280

## Ingredients:

- 2 large eggs
- 2 bacon slices
- 1 large halved and seeded plum tomato
- 2 tbsp chopped mixed herbs

- 2 tbsp grated parmesan cheese
- Salt and pepper

## Preparation:

| 1. | Season the tomato halves with salt and pepper. Then put half of the herbs in each cup. |
|----|---|
| 2. | Crack one egg into each cup. Sprinkle some salt, pepper and cheese over it. |
| 3. | Place bacon on the baking sheet. |
| 4. | Bake it in an oven preheated at 450-degrees Fahrenheit for 7 minutes. |
| 5. | Serve with a topping of bacon. |

*Lunch:* **Black Bean Soup**

*Dinner:* **Tamarind Fish and Okra**

*Breakfast:* **Apple Tea**

*Lunch:* **Grilled Chicken with Quinoa and Chipotle**

### Serves 4/31 min

Net carbs: 28% (25g/0.9oz) | Fiber: 10% (9g/0.3oz) | Fat: 21% (19g/0.7oz) | Protein: 40% (36g/1.27oz) | kcal: 450

## Ingredients:

- 1 lb boneless chicken breast
- 1 diced ripe avocado
- 2 cups shredded lettuce
- 2 cups cooked quinoa
- 1 cup rinsed pinto beans
- ¼ cup shredded cheddar cheese
- ¼ cup salsa
- 1 tbsp extra-virgin olive oil
- 1 tbsp chopped chipotle peppers
- ½ tsp ground cumin
- ½ tsp garlic powder
- ¼ tsp salt

## Preparation:

| | |
|---|---|
| **1.** | Combine oil, cumin, garlic powder and chipotles. |
| **2.** | Season the chicken breasts with salt and grill it for 5 minutes. Rub with the chipotle mix and turn the piece. Continue grilling in this mode for 5 more minutes. |
| **3.** | After they are done and have cooled down, chop them accordingly. |
| **4.** | Combine the chicken, quinoa, lettuce, beans, avocado, salsa and cheese. Serve fresh. |

*Dinner:* **Taco Meatloaf**

*Breakfast:* **PBJ Oatmeal Cups**

*Lunch:* **Tijuana Torta**

*Dinner:* **South Pacific Shrimp**

### Serves 4/45 min

Net carbs: 2% (7g/0.3oz) | Fiber: 3% (1g/0.03oz) | Fat: 13% (4g/0.14oz) | Protein: 58% (17g/0.6oz) | kcal: 135

## Ingredients:

- 1 lb deveined shrimp
- ½ cup coconut milk
- 2 minced jalapeno peppers
- 1 minced garlic clove
- 1 tsp extra-virgin olive oil4 cups baby spinach

- ½ cup diced tomato
- 1 tbsp brown sugar
- ¼ cup lemon juice
- 2 tsp soy sauce
- 1 tsp minced ginger

## Preparation:

| | |
|---|---|
| **1.** | Mix brown sugar, coconut milk, soy sauce, lemon juice, garlic, ginger and chilis. Add shrimp to coat and let it marinate in the refrigerator for 15 minutes. Then drain it to reserve the marinade. |
| **2.** | Cook the marinated shrimp at medium-high heat. Remove it from heat and place on a plate. |
| **3.** | Cook spinach and tomato in the same pan. Add the marinade and let it simmer for a couple of minutes. Bring back the shrimp to this pan and cook. |

*Breakfast:* **Banana-Almond Smoothie**

### Serves 2/5 min

Net carbs: 37% (26g/0.9oz) | Fiber: 7% (5g/0.18oz) | Fat: 25% (18g/0.6oz) | Protein: 30% (21g/0.74oz) | kcal: 330

## Ingredients:

- ½ banana cut into pieces
- ½ cup ice
- ¼ cup coconut water
- ¼ cup Greek yogurt
- 2 tbsp vanilla whey protein powder
- 1 tbsp almond butter
- 2 tbsp hulled hemp seeds

## Preparation:

| 1. | Blend all the Ingredients for at least a minute. Serve fresh. |
|----|---|

*Lunch:* **Zucchini Chili-Cheddar Mash**

*Dinner:* **Chicken Chili Rellenos**

*Breakfast:* **Light Smoothie**

*Lunch:* **Chili-lime Veggie Noodles**

### Serves 5/33 min

Net carbs: 54% (40g/1.4oz) | Fiber: 13% (10g/0.35oz) | Fat: 12% (9g/0.3oz) | Protein: 20% (15g/0.5oz) | kcal: 340

## Ingredients:

- 8 oz cooked whole-wheat spaghetti
- 4 large beaten eggs
- 2 sliced bell peppers
- 1 bunch of sliced scallions
- 6 cups sliced green cabbage
- 3 cups sliced mushroom caps

- 1 tsp lime zest
- 3 tbsp soy sauce
- 2 tbsp chili-garlic sauce
- 2 tbsp lime juice
- 1½ tbsp canola oil
- 1 tbsp light brown sugar

## Preparation:

| | |
|---|---|
| **1.** | Mix lime juice, lime zest, soy sauce, chili-garlic sauce, sherry and brown sugar. |
| **2.** | On a pan coated with 1 tsp oil, cook an omelet with the eggs. When it cools down, cut them into several strips. |
| **3.** | Fry the mushrooms and bell peppers using rest of the oil. Stir the cabbage and scallions into the mixture. |
| **4.** | When the vegetables become tender, add the noodles, chili-lime sauce and omelet strips. |

*Dinner:* **Salmon with Mango Sauce**

*Breakfast:* **Berry Blast**

*Lunch:* **BBQ Chicken Salad**

*Dinner:* **Fish Tacos with Lime and Mango**

### Serves 8/30 min

Net carbs: 37% (30g/1.1oz) | Fiber: 8% (6g/0.2oz) | Fat: 16% (13g/0.46oz) | Protein: 39% (31g/1.1oz) | kcal: 370

## Ingredients:

- 2 lbs skinless sole
- 6 oz crumbled cotija cheese
- 16 tortillas
- 2 sliced limes
- ½ sliced onion
- 6 cups shredded cabbage
- 2 cups chopped mangoes
- ¾ cup sour cream
- 2 tsp canola oil
- ½ tsp salt
- 1 tsp cumin seeds
- ½ tsp garlic powder
- ¼ tsp black pepper

## Preparation:

| | |
|---|---|
| **1.** | Season the fish with ¼ tsp salt, pepper and garlic powder. With a topping of lime slices, bake it for 7 minutes. Flake the fish coarsely. |
| **2.** | Cook cumin seeds, onion and rest of the salt in a skillet. When you get the familiar fragrance, stir in the cabbage and keep cooking. |
| **3.** | Fill the tortillas with the cabbage mixture first. Then top them with the fish, cheese, mangoes and sour cream. |

*Breakfast:* **Cafe Mocha Smoothie**

Serves 1/5 min

## Ingredients:

- ¾ cup chilled brewed coffee
- ½ cup whole milk
- ½ cup ice
- 1 diced banana
- 1 scoop chocolate whey protein powder
- 1 tbsp cocoa powder

## Preparation:

| 1. | Blend all the Ingredients for about a minute and serve immediately. |
|---|---|

*Lunch:* **Chicken Lettuce Wraps**

*Dinner:* **Turkey Skewers with Coconut**

*Breakfast:* **Almond and Bacon Pancakes**

*Lunch:* **Veggie Avocado-Bean Wrap**

### Serves 4/25 min

Net carbs: 41% (30g/1.1oz) | Fiber: 18% (13g/0.46oz) | Fat: 23% (17g/0.6oz) | Protein: 17% (12g/0.4oz) | kcal: 345

## Ingredients:

- 15-oz rinsed white beans
- 4 whole-wheat wraps
- 1 ripe avocado
- 1 shredded carrot
- 2 cups shredded cabbage
- ½ cup shredded cheddar cheese

- 2 tbsp cider vinegar
- 2 tbsp minced onion
- ¼ cup chopped cilantro
- 1 tbsp canola oil
- 2 tsp chopped chipotle chili
- ¼ tsp salt

## Preparation:

| | |
|---|---|
| **1.** | Combine carrot, cabbage and cilantro in one bowl. Mix chipotle chili, vinegar, oil and salt separately. Then use it to toss the vegetable mixture. |
| **2.** | In another bowl, mash avocado and white beans. Add cheese and onion while continuing to stir. |
| **3.** | Distribute the avocado-bean mix and the veggie mix evenly among the wraps. |

*Dinner:* **Chicken Breasts with Almond Cream Sauce**

*Breakfast:* **Breakfast Burrito**

*Lunch:* **Miso Beef Ramen**

*Dinner:* **Chipotle Beef Tacos with Pico de Gallo**

### Serves 8/40 min

Net carbs: 31% (20g/0.7oz) | Fiber: 6% (4g/0.14oz) | Fat: 19% (12g/0.4oz) | Protein: 43% (27g/0.95oz) | kcal: 320

## Ingredients:

- 2 lbs lean ground beef
- 16 white corn tortillas
- ¼ cup cider vinegar
- 2 cups chopped tomatoes
- 1 tsp ground cumin
- 1 cup chopped avocado
- ¾ cup beef broth
- 1 cup chopped onion

- ½ cup snipped cilantro
- ⅓ cup unsalted tomato paste
- 1 tsp dried oregano
- ½ tsp black pepper
- ½ tsp ground chipotle chili pepper
- ¼ tsp red pepper
- ¼ tsp salt

## Preparation:

| | |
|---|---|
| **1.** | Mix avocado, tomato, cilantro and red pepper to prepare the pico de gallo. |
| **2.** | Cook onion and garlic for 5 minutes on a coated non-stick skillet. Then blend it with beef broth, tomato paste, vinegar, oregano, cumin, pepper and salt to create a smooth mixture. |
| **3.** | Cook the ground beef until it turns brown. After draining it, add the onion mixture and cook again. Let it simmer for a while. |
| **4.** | Serve the meat inside tortillas with the pico de gallo. |

*Breakfast:* **Eggs with Grilled Asparagus**

### Serves 1/15 min

Net carbs: 10% (6g/0.2oz) | Fiber: 5% (3g/0.1oz) | Fat: 43% (25g/0.9oz) | Protein: 41% (24g/0.85oz) | kcal: 350

## Ingredients:

- 7 trimmed asparagus spears
- 2 large eggs
- ½ diced onion
- 3 tbsp grated parmesan cheese
- 2 tsp olive oil
- Salt and pepper

## Preparation:

| | |
|---|---|
| 1. | Grill asparagus and onion until they both get tender. |
| 2. | Chop the grilled onion and asparagus. Combine and season them with salt and pepper. |
| 3. | Cook the eggs with salt and pepper seasonings for 3 minutes. |
| 4. | Spread the asparagus and onion hash on the serving plate. Place eggs on top with a sprinkle of cheese. |

*Lunch:* **Radish and Asparagus Salad**

*Dinner:* **Baked Shrimp Enchilada**

*Breakfast:* **Blueberry Muffin Parfait**

*Lunch:* **BBQ Portobello Quesadillas**

### Serves 2/45 min

Net carbs: 56% (40g/1.41oz) | Fiber: 7% (5g/0.18oz) | Fat: 20% (14g/0.5oz) | Protein: 16% (12g/0.4oz) | kcal: 325

## Ingredients:

- ½ lb trimmed and diced portobello mushroom caps
- 2 whole-wheat tortillas
- ½ minced chipotle chili
- ½ diced onion

- ¼ cup BBQ sauce
- 6 tbsp shredded cheese
- 1 tbsp canola oil
- 1½ tsp cider vinegar
- 1½ tsp tomato paste

## Preparation:

| | |
|---|---|
| **1.** | Mix BBQ sauce, chipotle, tomato paste and vinegar. |
| **2.** | Cook the mushrooms with 2 tsp of oil for a while. Then add the onions and keep stirring until the mushrooms start to turn brown. |
| **3.** | Take out the cooked vegetables and toss it with the BBQ sauce mix. |
| **4.** | Fill up each tortilla with 3 tbsp cheese and one quarter of the vegetable mix. Fold and press each filled tortilla to make the quesadillas. |
| **5.** | Cook the quesadillas in a pan coated with 1 tsp oil. Make sure both of its sides is brown. |

*Dinner:* **Beef Bean Verde**

*Breakfast:* **Baked Ham and Cheese**

*Lunch:* **Radish and Asparagus Salad**

*Dinner:* **Vietnamese Shrimp Lettuce Wraps**

### Serves 4/37 min

Net carbs: 20% (7g/0.3oz) | Fiber: 6% (2g/0.07oz) | Fat: 11% (4g/0.14oz) | Protein: 62% (22g/0.78oz) | kcal: 150

## Ingredients:

- 1 lb deveined shrimp
- 1 sliced red chili
- 1 head butter lettuce
- ½ cup julienned carrot
- ½ cup julienned mango
- ½ cup julienned radish
- ½ cup cilantro leaves
- 2 tbsp lemon juice
- 1 tbsp canola oil
- 1 tbsp fish sauce
- 1 tsp brown sugar

## Preparation:

| | |
|---|---|
| **1.** | Mix brown sugar, lemon juice, chili and fish sauce. Use this mixture to coat a combination of mango, carrot and radishes. |
| **2.** | Cook the shrimp for 4 minutes on a hot skillet. |
| **3.** | Combine the shrimp and the mango mix. Let it sit for a while. |
| **4.** | Serve with cilantro and lettuce leaves. |

*Breakfast:* **Cuban Sandwich**

### Serves 1/20 min

Net carbs: 54% (45g/1.58oz) | Fiber: 7% (6g/0.2oz) | Fat: 10% (9g/0.3oz) | Protein: 28% (24g/0.85oz) | kcal: 390

## Ingredients:

- 2 oz sliced lean pork loin
- 2 oz whole-wheat baguette, halved
- 1 slice of baked ham
- 1 tbsp Greek yogurt
- 1 trimmed Portobello mushroom,
- gills discarded
- 1 sliced red onion
- 1 tbsp light mayonnaise
- 1 tbsp sweet pickle relish
- ½ tsp olive oil

## Preparation:

| 1. | Cook the combination of mushroom and onion in oil for 10 minutes. Cut the mushroom in half when it's done. |
| 2. | Take a halved baguette on one side. Layer it with yogurt, mayo and relish. Use pork, ham, mushroom halves and onion slices as toppings. Complete the sandwich with the other half of baguette. |
| 3. | Press the sandwich as per need and cook for a minute. |

*Lunch:* **Veggie Tabbouleh**

*Dinner:* **Pork and Soba Noodles**

*Breakfast:* **Boiled Eggs and Sweet Potatoes**

*Lunch:* **Peanut Noodles with Chicken and Vegetables**

### Serves 6/33 min

Net carbs: 38% (30g/1.1oz) | Fiber: 10% (8g/0.3oz) | Fat: 16% (13g/0.46oz) | Protein: 35% (27g/0.95oz) | kcal: 375

## Ingredients:

- 1 lb cooked and shredded boneless chicken breasts
- 12 oz of vegetable mix
- 8 oz whole-wheat spaghetti
- 2 tsp minced garlic

- ½ cup peanut butter
- 2 tbsp soy sauce
- 1 tsp minced ginger
- 1 tsp chili-garlic sauce

## Preparation:

| | |
|---|---|
| **1.** | Mix soy sauce, chili-garlic sauce, peanut butter, ginger and garlic. |
| **2.** | Cook the pasta with vegetables and then drain the threads. |
| **3.** | Stir the remaining liquid in the pasta pot to the peanut sauce. Use it to toss pasta, chicken and vegetables. |

*Dinner:* **Tamarind Fish and Okra**

*Breakfast:* **Quinoa Porridge**

*Lunch:* **Bean Tacos with Green Salsa**

*Dinner:* **Korean Turkey Burgers**

### Serves 4/30 min

Net carbs: 35% (25g/0.9oz) | Fiber: 7% (5g/0.18oz) | Fat: 17% (12g/0.4oz) | Protein: 40% (28g/1oz) | kcal: 340

## Ingredients:

- 1 lb ground turkey
- 4 toasted hamburger buns
- 3 sliced scallions
- 2 sliced cucumber
- 1 cup kimchi
- 2 tbsp low-fat mayonnaise
- 8 tsp chili paste
- 1 tsp toasted sesame oil

## Preparation:

| | |
|---|---|
| **1.** | Gently combine the turkey, sesame oil, scallions and 5 tsps. of chili paste to form 4 burger patties of equal thickness. |
| **2.** | Grill them all and then let them cool down. Then place them inside the burger buns. |
| **3.** | Mix mayonnaise and rest of the chili paste. Use this as topping on each burger along with cucumber slices and kimchi. |

*Breakfast:* **Shakshuka**

### Serves 4/1 hour 25 min

Net carbs: 25% (14g/0.5oz) | Fiber: 9% (5g/0.18oz) | Fat: 42% (24g/0.85oz) | Protein: 23% (13g/0.46oz) | kcal: 333

## Ingredients:

- 4 large eggs
- 3 lbs plum tomatoes, diced
- 3 garlic cloves (2 sliced, 1 chopped)
- 2 chopped large chilis
- 3 tbsp chopped parsley
- ½ tsp ground pepper
- ½ cup shredded feta cheese
- 1 chopped onion
- ¾ tsp salt
- ⅓ cup chopped basil
- 4 tbsp extra-virgin olive oil
- 1 tsp ground cumin

## Preparation:

| | |
|---|---|
| **1.** | Mix the tomatoes, sliced garlic cloves, onion, some parsley, 3 tbsp oil, pinch of salt and pepper. Spread this combination on a baking sheet and roast for 40 minutes. |
| **2.** | Heat up a skillet with the rest of oil. Cook the chopped garlic and chilis for a couple of minutes. Then stir in the cumin, tomato mixture, basil and rest of salt. Keep cooking until most of the tomatoes have broken down. |
| **3.** | Use your spoon to create four caves in this mixture. Crack one egg in each cave and sprinkle the remaining pepper over them. Cook with the lid on for 7 minutes. |
| **4.** | Spread the feta cheese on top and cook for 2 more minutes. |
| **5.** | Serve with parsley. |

*Lunch:* **Black Bean Soup**

*Dinner:* **Taco Meatloaf**

*Breakfast:* **PBJ Oatmeal Cups**

*Lunch:* **Chicken Cucumber Noodles Salad**

### Serves 12/45 min

Net carbs: 31% (15g/0.5oz) | Fiber: 6% (3g/0.1oz) | Fat: 25% (12g/0.4oz) | Protein: 38% (18g/0.6oz) | kcal: 240

## Ingredients:

- 1½ lb cooked and sliced boneless chicken
- 8 oz cooked egg noodles
- 2 diced red bell peppers
- 1 sliced cucumber
- 1 trimmed head romaine lettuce
- 1 cup peanut butter
- 2 tbsp toasted sesame oil
- 1 cup sliced scallions
- ¾ cup rice vinegar
- ¼ cup chopped cilantro
- 2 tbsp dry sherry
- 2 tbsp soy sauce
- 1 tbsp chili sauce
- Salt and pepper

## Preparation:

| | |
|---|---|
| **1.** | Mix sherry, peanut butter, sesame oil and vinegar first. Then add the scallions, cilantro, chili sauce and soy sauce to prepare the dressing. |
| **2.** | Combine the noodles, chicken, lettuce, bell peppers and cucumber. Toss it with the dressing. |
| **3.** | Season with salt and pepper. Serve fresh. |

*Dinner:* **Chicken Chili Rellenos**

*Breakfast:* **Light Smoothie**

*Lunch:* **Tijuana Torta**

*Dinner:* **Ceviche Avocados**

### Serves 6/1 hour

Net carbs: 13% (5g/0.18oz) | Fiber: 18% (7g/0.3oz) | Fat: 44% (17g/0.6oz) | Protein: 24% (9g/0.3oz) | kcal: 220

## Ingredients:

- 6 oz chopped cooked shrimp
- 3 ripe avocados
- 1 chopped jalapeno
- ¼ cup chopped tomato
- 1 tsp sugar

- ¼ cup chopped cucumber
- 2 tbsp chopped cilantro
- 1 tbsp extra-virgin olive oil
- ¼ tsp salt
- Juice of 4 lemons

## Preparation:

| | |
|---|---|
| **1.** | Mix the lemon juice and sugar until the latter dissolves. Use this to coat the shrimp which then needs to stay in the refrigerator for 45 minutes. |
| **2.** | Drain the refrigerated shrimp. Combine it with oil, cucumber, tomato, jalapeno, cilantro and salt. |
| **3.** | Cut avocados in half and pit it. Fill up each half with the shrimp mixture. |

*Breakfast:* **Scrambled Eggs**

### Serves 1/10 min

Net carbs: 37% (20g/0.7oz) | Fiber: 6% (3g/0.1oz) | Fat: 24% (13g/0.46oz) | Protein: 32% (17g/0.6oz) | kcal: 275

## Ingredients:

♦ 2 large eggs, beaten

♦ 2 corn tortillas

♦ 1 tbsp salsa

♦ 1 tbsp shredded cheese

♦ 1 tsp cilantro

## Preparation:

| | |
|---|---|
| **1.** | Cook the eggs on a non-stick skillet. |
| **2.** | Add cheese and salsa in the end. |
| **3.** | Fill up the tortillas with this mixture and use cilantro for topping. |

*Lunch:* **Zucchini Chili-Cheddar Mash**

*Dinner:* **Salmon with Mango Sauce**

*Breakfast:* **Almond and Bacon Pancakes**

*Lunch:* **Lentil and Eggplant Salad**

### Serves 4/45 min

Net carbs: 56% (65g/2.3oz) | Fiber: 15% (17g/0.6oz) | Fat: 17% (20g/0.7oz) | Protein: 12% (14g/0.5oz) | kcal: 510

## Ingredients:

- 2 diced eggplants
- 2 diced ripe mangoes
- 2 bunches of chopped scallions
- 4 cups romaine lettuce
- 1 2/3 cups cooked lentils
- 2½ tsp curry powder
- ⅓ cup lime juice
- ¼ cup chopped cilantro

- ¼ cup chopped cashews
- ¼ cup honey
- ¼ cup salsa
- 4 tbsp olive oil
- 2½ tsp chili powder
- ¼ tsp ground pepper
- ¼ tsp salt

## Preparation:

| | |
|---|---|
| **1.** | Mix 2 tsp chili powder, 2 tsp curry powder with 1 tbsp oil. Use this to toss the eggplant cubes. Bake it for 15 minutes. |
| **2.** | Combine rest of the oil and both powders with honey, salsa, lime juice, salt and pepper. Then use it to toss a mixture of the roasted eggplant, scallions and lentils. |
| **3.** | Serve it with toppings of nuts, mango, lettuce and cilantro. |

*Dinner:* **Turkey Skewers with Coconut**

*Breakfast:* **Blueberry Muffin Parfait**

*Lunch:* **Radish and Asparagus Salad**

*Dinner:* **Cod Pomodoro**

## Serves 4/20 min

Net carbs: 26% (14g/0.5oz) | Fiber: 6% (3g/0.1oz) | Fat: 11% (6g/0.2oz) | Protein: 56% (29g/1oz) | kcal: 232

## Ingredients:

- ◆ 28 oz crushed tomatoes
- ◆ 1 chopped shallot
- ◆ 4 cod fillets
- ◆ 1 tbsp olive oil
- ◆ 3 minced garlic cloves
- ◆ ½ cup chopped basil
- ◆ 1 tsp honey
- ◆ Salt and pepper

## Preparation:

| | |
|---|---|
| **1.** | Season the fish fillets with pepper and salt. Then cook them in hot oil for 2-4 minutes per side. Transfer it to a plate. |
| **2.** | In the same skillet, sauté shallots and garlic until they get tender. Stir in the honey and crushed tomatoes. Let it simmer for a while. |
| **3.** | Return the fillets to this skillet, along with basil. Simmer for a couple of minutes. Serve warm. |

The opinions and ideas of the author contained in this publication are designed to educate the reader in an informative and helpful manner. While we accept that the instructions will not suit every reader, it is only to be expected that the recipes might not gel with everyone. Use the book responsibly and at your own risk. This work with all its contents, does not guarantee correctness, completion, quality or correctness of the provided information. Always check with your medical practitioner should you be unsure whether to follow a low carb eating plan. Misinformation or misprints cannot be completely eliminated. Human error is real!

Printed in Poland
by Amazon Fulfillment
Poland Sp. z o.o., Wrocław